KEYS TO INTERMITTENT FASTING

When You Are Ready To Change Your Life . . .

AMINE SALHI

TABLE OF CONTENTS

INTRODUCTION: WHAT IS FASTING?

The dietary phenomenon we call 'fasting' – the voluntary self-denial of food, drink, or both for a period of time – has a long history throughout the evolution of the human species, worldwide. Fasting has generally been used as a tool for achieving distinct results with regard to health, religion, ritual, or for ethical and aesthetic reasons.

Fasting is considered a behavioral phenomenon because eating sustains life and provides energy. All creatures from microscopic amoeba to huge whales must eat. For animals in the wild, the very act of hunting for food is a perpetual pursuit with no "days off." Few mammals, fish, oceanic or amphibious creatures, birds or insects are able or inclined to store food. For them, the search for something to eat in order to maintain health, energy and life itself, consumes many hours of every day or night.

Hibernating mammals exhibit a pattern of gaining huge amounts of fatty weight in the Spring, Summer and Fall that will nourish them as they sleep through the cold and barren winter. By Spring, when these creatures emerge from hibernation, they will have lost considerable weight, awakening only to start the seasonal cycle once more.

Animals and other creatures do not willingly refuse food or water.

Although humans approaching the end of life commonly opt to refuse food and drink, this oft-voluntary action is not seen as a form of fasting, but instead, a conscious decision aimed to hasten death and to end suffering.

In this vein, animals also have been known to follow suit. Pet owners often know the end is near when their animal companion starts to exhibit a distinct reluctance to eat and drink.

Refusing to eat and/or hydrate is *not* normal behavior.

THE HISTORY OF FASTING

From its earliest times, fasting has been a uniquely human behavior. Unless they are literally at death's door, animals do not willingly refuse food – and certainly never for ideological, spiritual, esoteric or religious reasons.

The voluntary abstention of food through fasting is a phenomenon that has been avidly pursued by ascetics, by indigenous 'medicine men' and pagan priestesses, and by holy hermits in pursuit of visionary experiences. Fasting has been used by members of religious orders, and by their followers, as well by millions of people practicing any one of the many world religions that require fasting as a form of penance for sins of omission or commission, and as a means of spiritual cleansing.

While fasting has been criticized from its origin as being abnormal and unhealthful, the opposite has also been true. Indeed, early Greek physicians lauded the benefits of fasting.

Existing records from the ancient world reveal that abstinence from some or all food, for a certain period of time – whether complete, or partial – was a practice utilized by the cultures of Babylon and

Assyria, Greece, Tome, Palestine, India, Persia, China. Cuneiform and hieroglyphic writing from Mesopotamia and Egypt reference fasting as an important element of their religious rituals.

Pythagoras of Samos, the famed Greek political and religious teacher, philosopher, and noted mathematician, also espoused the practice of fasting, as did the 14th century Dominican ascetic, St. Catherine of Siena, who advocated for rigorous fasting.

In other cultures, warriors fasted in preparation of going to war, while other employed fasting as a part of "coming of age" trials that ended in elaborate ceremonies.

Indigenous North Americans used to fast to train their bodies to experience less deprivation in meager times. When a youth was old enough to be initiated into the tribe, the young man would be sent into the wilderness for a period of days, alone, during which time he underwent a sustained fast of one to four days, often without access to fluids. Upon his return, food was reintroduced slowly, until his system could once again accommodate a full meal. Fasting was also a medium of communication with the forces that exist beyond the five senses, inducing visions, hallucinations, and extraordinary dreams. Fasting was considered a method of acquiring occult power or negotiating with spirits, and Tribal shamans fasted frequently as part of their duties and to maintain their spiritual powers. Tribal chiefs often ordered the entire tribe to fast, in order to avert disasters such as famine or other catastrophes, and to appeal for plentiful hunts.

Fasting has also been central to the religious ceremonies of every known religion on earth, as it is thought to remove the spirit for a period of time from its mortal ties, needs and concerns, in an effort to purify the soul. The Incas of Peru and Native Americans of Mexico both appeased their gods through penitential fasting. Apart from its religious connections, fasting has long been associated with magic. It is associated with certain forms of discipline, and as a form of exhibition to garner public attention to a cause.

Through history, women have fasted in order to maintain their figures – or because peculiarities of dress or tight corsets left no room for food. In fact, conventional manners of the times dictated that "ladies" were to eat sparingly lest they appear "unseemly," or gluttonous.

During the 19th Century, therapeutic fasting under medical supervision came into vogue, to either treat or prevent a variety of illnesses as a part of that era's "Natural Hygiene Movement."

In the 20th Century, the "hunger strike" was used by individuals and groups of people to attract notoriety and publicity for certain causes. Political activist Bobby Sands and his comrades use hunger strikes in North Ireland, following on the heels of civil unrest within the heavily divided country.

The hunger strike as a form of fasting, has been used as a political weapon for centuries, by and on behalf of political prisoners worldwide, and even by conscientious objectors protesting the military draft during the Vietnam War. One of the most renowned modern practitioner of fasting was Mohandas Ghandi, better known in the West by the honorific title, Mahatma (meaning 'Great Soul'), a name bestowed on him by his followers in India during his struggle to attain India's freedom from the British.

Ghandi repeatedly undertook fasts and encouraged his followers to join him in such non-violent demonstrations against the Crown.

Types of Fasting

While some rules for fasting are very specific and religious oriented, others are far less structured and be without a specific purpose.

Fasting that requires abstinence from both food *and* drink is usually done for ritualistic or religious purposes, or in advance of medical procedures which require a stomach and/or intestinal tract, devoid of content.

Most fasts encourage frequent hydration and allow a person to imbibe lots of water and unlimited quantities of clear liquids or non-caloric beverages such as water, unsugared tea, and black coffee.

Fasts can last for hours, days, or weeks at a time, and can be of short duration, or be undertaken just during a certain period of the day. Forms of fasting may require complete abstinence, partial abstinence, or some manner of intermittent abstinence.

When a fast demands abstinence from *all* food and drink, it is known as an 'absolute' or 'dry' fast.

Criticism of fasting, long considered 'unnatural,' and disruptive to social order, has ranged from challenge throughout history by religious leaders faulting fasting as hypocritical when used in lieu of true repentance for sins, to more modern complaints from psychologists and doctors who decry the practice of long-term and rigorous fasting as a hazard to both mental and physical health.

Modern society has also taken issue with fasting for health related reasons, eschewing eschews rigorous fasts and long-term total abstinence where even water is refused/ As a result, selective, short term fasts are more commonly preferred.

Despite the many warnings and criticisms, and the reality that many people remain dubious as to the acceptability of fasting, there is no medical evidence to support the notion that, for the average person, intermittent fasting is a medically dangerous practice.

There are obviously exceptions. If you take prescription medication or have medical problems, then you should consult your doctor before beginning a fasting routine for any reason.

Intermittent fasting (IF) differs from most forms of caloric restriction. IF doesn't identify the foods you should eat or set calorie limits; rather, IF establishes the time frames or intervals within which you should eat.

Also known as intermittent energy restriction, intermittent fasting is an umbrella term for a number of meal timing schedules that alternate between periods of voluntary fasting and non-fasting over a given expanse of time.

Fasting for Healing - Ancient Origins of the Practice

"Everyone has a physician inside him or her; we just have to help it in its work. The natural healing force within each one of us is the greatest force in getting well. Our food should be our medicine. Our medicine should be our food. But to eat when you are sick is to feed your sickness."

Hippocrates

"Fasting is the greatest remedy - the physician within."

Parcelsus

"Humans live on one-quarter of what they eat; on the other three-quarters lives their doctor."

Egyptian pyramid inscription

Based upon ancient history, fasting is one of the oldest healing traditions known to man.

One of the fathers of modern medicine, Hippocrates of Cos (c 460 - c 370 BC) both championed and personally prescribed the practice of fasting as a treatment for many ills.

He also recommended the consumption of apple cider vinegar – a tried and true health remedy that has stood the test of time and is still a valid and frequent wellness recommendation today. Fellow Greek scholar, Plutarch (cAD46 – cAD 120) echoed similar sentiments in opining that man was better off fasting than using medicine.

The revitalizing and rejuvenating power of fasting were readily recognized by healers in the ancient world who advocated for fasting, both as a healing therapy and for the general health and mental acuity of an individual. Another godfather of Western medicine, Paracelsus, believed that the healing qualities of fasting unleashed the body's ability to heal itself, a fact which has been further supported by modern research. Clearly the ancient Greeks were in tune with nature and developed many of their healing techniques and philosophies from their observation of natural processes and behaviors.

For instance, most animals refrain from eating when they are sick, and humans do as well. Both instinctively fast when sick, or dying, which can also manifest in an illness-related form of anorexia in response to certain debilitating health conditions. Even American thinker, publisher and Founding Father, Benjamin Franklin (1706-1790) noted the correlation between fasting and health, where he related that '*the best of all medicines is resting and fasting.*'

Not surprisingly, devotees of the ancient practice of fasting maintain that it results in both spiritual and physical renewal and increased vigor. More recently, such notions are supported by modern practitioners like Herbert Shelton (1895-1985), who supervised the individual fasts of more than 40,000 people during the past century. With respect to such experience, he posited that noted that fasting must be recognized as a fundamental and radical process that is older than any other mode of caring for the sick.

Fasting for Religious Reasons

Fasting has also been practiced for centuries as a religious observance, since before recorded history. Fasting that is part of a religious ritual may involve the repetition of certain prayers or practices, as well as particular rituals and ceremonies.

Recorded religious history has made frequent references to fasting among both non-Christian and Christian practitioners. There are many specific references to fasting in the both the Old and New Testament books of the Bible. Fasting in religious practice often involves deliberate abstinence from gratification by rejecting food for a period of time. This is done, however, in order to achieve greater spiritual communication with the Almighty, and such fasts are often quite rigorous, and may involve deprivation of all fluids, including water. This type of fast is called an 'absolute fast' or 'dry fasting,' is more commonly known as total abstinence of all food and liquid for a defined period of time.

The Gospels of Matthew, Mark and Luke further relate the temptation of Christ as a biblical narrative, for after his baptism by John the Baptist, the Gospels tell us that Jesus retreated into the Judaean Desert and engaged in a rigorous fast for 40 days and 40 nights. This would appear to have been an absolute, or dry fast.

For reasons that this book will address in subsequent chapters, fasting has gained in popularity in recent years. People are beginning to understand – after thousands of years during which humankind has fasted primarily for religious reasons – that the act of fasting benefits far more than just the human spirit. It offers individuals who fast, a veritable cornucopia of positive physical results that are cognitive, curative, aesthetic, and contribute to overall health maintenance.

Early Christian writers echoed Old Testament prophets who often dismissed the value of religious fasts, criticizing them as empty and deceptive demonstrations employed by sinners to divert attention from their immoral activities. Despite such criticism, religious fasts continue to be observed by Jews, Christians, Muslims, Hindus, Confucianists, Taoists, Jainists, and those who adhere to many other faiths, including Tibetan Buddhists.

The energy depletion which results from long fasts suspended or reduced normal physical activity, can result in a state of quiescence described as being symbolic of death, or akin to the human state immediately preceding birth.

Pagan and primitive ceremonies often incorporated fasting around fertility rituals, and in ceremonies organized at the vernal and autumn equinoxes. It is said that these ceremonies endured for centuries, often masquerading under other names as the societal faiths changed over time.

A number of religious scholars have connected these early rites to the Jewish use of unleavened bread when celebrating the spring festival of Passover (Pesach), and claim that traces of ancient ritual fasting are demonstrated by the Lenten fasts observed by Christians in their spiritual preparation for the celebration of Easter.

The Jewish use of fasting as a form of purification and penance is a form of religious observation practiced annually on Yom Kippur, the Day of Atonement, since its establishment by Moses. Neither food nor drink is permitted on this sacred day.

Among early Christians, fasting was also associated with penance and with purification (Mark 9:29; Matthew 6:16), and during the first two centuries of the current era, the Catholic Church established fasts as a voluntary means of preparing oneself spiritually for the sacraments of baptism and Holy Communion, as well as in preparation for ordination to the priesthood. The practice was voluntary until later, when fasting became obligatory. Subsequently a series of feast days and fasting days were added to the Church calendar, and in the 6th century the Lenten fast of only 40 hours (the time Jesus was thought to have spent in the tomb) was extended a the period of 40 days – the length of time Christ fasted in the desert. Only one meal was permitted to be eaten during those 40 days of Lent.

On the heels of the Reformation, Protestant churches continued the practice of Lenten fast, although it was made optional in certain cases. With the evolution of Protestantism stricter followers of the faith, such as the Puritans, rejected the Church festivals that had originated with Catholicism, as well as the fasts dictated by the Church of Rome. The Easter Orthodox Catholic Church rigorously observes its fasts, although its calendar differs significantly from that of the Roman Catholic Church.

Currently, fasting in the Roman Catholic Church involves abstinence from food prior to taking Holy Communion, but permits water. Total abstinence is voluntary. Currently, only two days in the Roman Catholic Church remain as fast days: Ash Wednesday and Good Friday. Among non-Catholics in the United States, fasting practices are observed by Lutherans and Episcopalians, Orthodox and Roman Catholics, and by Conservative Jews. In many instances, the requirements governing fasting have been relaxed, and exceptions have been made for individuals suffering from certain health conditions, such as diabetes, and for those taking certain medications that must be taken with a mead, as well as individuals in military service.

During the month of Ramadan, Muslims fast by day but can eat after dark. Their daily fasts during this holy month are a form of atonement for the sins of the past year.

Zoroastrianism is the only religion that prohibits fasting. All other religions have endorsed fasting as a form of penance, self-discipline, as evidence of self-control, and as a practice conducive to communications with the deity.

The many religions that incorporate fasting in their guidelines for the faithful do so for a variety of reasons. One common theme however, is that abstention from bodily nourishment brings the faithful closer to God, the Source, Allah or the Most High, and facilitates spiritual communication with the higher powers.

If you are not traditionally religious, you can still practice voluntary fasting as suits your needs or desires, whether a weekly, monthly, or annual fast lasting 24-hour hours, with intermittent fasting, or with a longer, three day fast during celebratory days of your choosing.

Currently the world's largest religions define fasting as follows:

Catholicism; Christianity: Modern fasting rules reduce the intake of food to a single large meal plus two smaller meals which, together, do not comprise an amount equivalent to the single large meal. Meat must be avoided, and no other food can be eaten. The requirement to avoid meat on Friday has been eliminated, but fasts are enforced in penitential periods such as Lent, the Wednesday, Friday and Saturday of each of the Ember weeks of the liturgical calendar: After 13 December (S. Lucia);

following Ash Wednesday (at the beginning of Lent); following Pentecost (also known as Whitsunday), and after the Exaltation of the Cross on September 14. These were established by Pope Gregory VII (1073-1085). The purpose of prayer and fasting during Ember days was to thank God for the gifts of nature, to teach men to utilize them moderately, and to succor the needy.

Fasting practices are now far less strict, the result of having been greatly in recent centuries. Fasts used to consist of one meal daily, eaten after the sun set, and consumption of eggs, dairy, meat, and alcohol was prohibited. During the final week of Lent, or Holy Week, that one meal consisted only of bread and water, with salt and herbs. In the 14th century the meal shifted to a full repast at lunch, with a snack at suppertime; a morning snack was added in the 19th century, and in the 20th century the fasting requirement was eliminated, and substituted with charitable works and prayer.

The Eastern Orthodox Church continues its fasting periods, permitting a single meal daily, but no animal products. The island of Crete, home to many Greek Orthodox Christians, boasts an extremely healthy population, with an average life expectancy of 81.4 years, and a large number of individuals still active into their 90s. Interestingly, Greek Orthodox Christians follow various religious fasts from 180 to 100 days of each year.

Mormonism: Mormons observe a 'Fast Sunday' on the first Sunday of each month that involves abstinence from two meals during a 24-hour period. On 'Fast Sunday' Church members publicly share personal testimonies.

Islam: Fasting is included as one of Islam's 'Five Pillars' – the others being prayer five times daily, charity, pilgrimage to Mecca, and a declaration of personal faith. Non-obligatory fast days occur every Monday and Thursday – or can be adopted every other day. A month-long period of mandatory fasting is called Ramadan, during which ingestion of food is forbidden from dawn to dark. After dark, there is no limit on the kinds or quantity that may be eaten. Alcohol is always prohibited in Islam, but smoking is also prohibited during times of fast. Fasting is forbidden on Islamic holy days that include a feast.

When beginning a religious fast in Islam, the individual must begin by setting a personal intention, which does not need to be made public. Should the fast bebroken for any reason, the period of the fast is extended by a day. If, however, the fast is broken through commission of a sexual act, one must free a slave (yes, slavery is still permitted by the Muslim religion and often by law as well, in countries where Islam is the majority religion), or fast by an additional two months, or feed or clothe 60 poor people.

Without setting a spiritual intention at the beginning of a fast, the practice is simply considered starving oneself. With the setting of a religious intention, fasting is undertaken to bring the faithful closer to Allah, to help control desire, to create a connection with others of the faith, and to create empathy with the less fortunate.

Judaism: Traditional Judaism recognizes six days through the year when one must fast, and can have neither food nor drink during a 24-hour period that lasts from sunset of the first day to sunset of the next.

During *Yom Kippur* and *Tisha B'Av*, an individual must also wash themselves and cannot wear anything made of leather, use perfume or cologne, or engage is sex. These restrictions do not apply to the other four fast days.

Buddhism: Buddhist monks and nuns following *Vijñāna* (Sanskrit) or vi*ññāna* (Pāli) - *Vinyana* to us Westerners – eschew all food after the noon meal, fasting for an extended period each day of the fast. However, this is not seen as a fast, but rather, a routine regime to aid meditation and support good health. Food is generally consumed in the morning hours. Eight other tenets of their religious practice forbid them from engaging in other activities: killing, stealing, engaging in sex (the monks and nuns are celibate), intoxication, 'wrong speech,' use of cosmetics, and music, dancing and singing. These are all activities that devout Buddhists refrain from throughout the year, while lay Buddhists routinely follow these rules on *Uposatha* days (in Sanskrit: *Upvasatha*), which are the weekly Sabbath days for all Buddhists, established and observed since 500 B.C.E., when the Buddha lived.

Hinduism: In Hindi, *vrata* is a term that means "vow, resolve, devotion." It refers to a practice of physical austerity, usually in matters regarding the consumption of food and drinks by the faithful in Hindu and Jain cultures. *Vrata* is an essential part of a pious observance involving certain obligations and includes absolute or partial fasting as well as prayers for love, health, fertility, long life or happiness for loved ones. Among the obligations of the *vrata* period are that individuals making the fast must remain celibate for the duration, must remain clean, abstain from meat, speak only the truth, perform specified rituals, and practice forbearance – exhibiting tolerance and restraint in the face of provocation. A *vrata* must never be left unfinished, once begun. Nor should another *vrata* be started before completing the first.

For Hindu practitioners, a strict fast demands absolute or 'dry' abstention of around 36 hours – no food and no water from sunset of the prior day to 48 minutes after the sun rises on the next. The *Ekadashi* are lunar phases occurring twice monthly, and fasting periods commence the sunset before to the sunrise after the *Ekadashi*. Then the deities each have their own fasting days: Where *Vishnu* requires fasting on a Thursday, *Shiva* demands a Monday fast.

Jainism: Jains practice a disciplined approach to eating 365 days of the year, never consuming food until they are fully satiated, and undertaking fast throughout the year. Jains are strict vegetarians, and religious fasting is widely observed. In the Jain religion, fasting is either an absolute, dry fast, or one that allows only water (which has been boiled to kill any and all microorganisms).

Spiritually oriented fasting is believed, in their religion, to check the physical demands of the body as it uplifts the soul. This also resolves and negative *karma* the individual may have accumulated through his or her actions or words. As they fast, they worship, meditate, read their scripture, perform charitable acts, and do whatever is required to serve the holy men and women – monks and nuns – who live among them. Most commonly, fasting is undertaken approximately twice a month on the 8th and 14th days of the moon's cycle, with long fasts of more than a week taking place during festivals, three times a year.

Conclusion: Jesus Christ, Buddha and the Muslim prophet Muhammed all advocated and practiced fasting in their own lives and saw it as a method of spiritual and physical healing that is deeply beneficial. Their followers continue the practice, and fasting for spiritual reasons continues in virtually all the religions of the world as a form of penitence and spiritual cleansing, to inspire deep thought and greater communication with their deities, and as a part of religious practices that intrinsically emphasizes control over bodily needs and desires while refreshing and stimulating the mind.

Fasting for Weight Loss

https://www.dietdoctor.com/intermittent-fasting

Intermittent fasting is also known as intermittent energy restriction, which is an umbrella term for a number of meal timing schedules that alternate between periods of voluntary fasting and non-fasting over a given expanse of time. Contrary to extremely strict fasting in which restrictions even disallow fluid intake, as is often required in religious practices, non-caloric and sometimes low-caloric drinks (usually referred to as 'clear liquids') can be taken during intermittent fasting.

A suggestion for anyone interested in adopting a practice of intermittent fasting is to try it for a month to see if an IF schedule works for you. Before diving in unprepared, start by following a high fat, high protein and low-carbohydrate diet in anticipation of adopting an IF fasting lifestyle. A low-carbohydrate ketogenic (Keto) diet is perfect to use in tandem with intermittent fasting, although other low-carbohydrate diets will also reduce your hunger, retrain your appetite, and so will make intermittent fasting easier. This kind of diet will also prevent you from bingeing on non-fasting days.

Even a low-carb diet may provide a degree of weight loss and type 2 diabetes reversal.

But be aware that if you overeat on your non-fast days, or if you continue eating simple carbohydrates, which readily turn into sugars in your system and provide instant energy, but soon leave you hungry, you may not lose weight with a fasting routine.

Examples of simple carbohydrates include food additives like white and brown sugars, corn syrup, glucose-fructose-sucrose, fruit juice concentrates, and common foods like baked goods, packaged cookies, sugary soda, and most common breakfast cereals.

Complex carbohydrates include fruits, vegetables, whole grains, legumes (beans and peas), oats, potatoes, and so forth. Complex carbohydrates have lots of fiber and are more filling; they take longer to digest and so satisfy hunger longer than simple carbs do.

What is intermittent fasting (IF), and how does it work? Intermittent fasting is an eating pattern, not a diet. With IF, you are making a conscious decision to intentionally skip meals on pre-determined days, or only eat within an 8-hour time frame, and fast for the other 16 hours every day. IF does not depend on calorie counting or continuous calorie reduction.

While there are a variety of methods to implement intermittent fasting, the different eating schedules that can be employed on an ongoing basis share a single concept: You eat normally during non-fasting periods but stick to a specific time frame for ingesting food, and fast over identified and planned days, or hours of the day.

Some types of IF diets are flexible and, rather than totally abstaining from all but water and clear, non-caloric fluids on fast days, suggest that you cut back instead to just 500-600 calories. For people fasting while under a doctor's care, or those who are on medications that must be taken with, before or after meals, this particular pattern is easier and medically safer than total abstinence.

In response to some Frequently Asked Questions (FAQ), please consider the following:

Limitations: Fasting is not a cakewalk. Skipping most of your week's normal calories for a few days a week and relying only on coffee, water and tea to maintain your fluid balance is frankly difficult, although if you stick to it, it does become easier over time. The key is to select a time frame that works for you, and fine tune your "feast day" eating beforehand.

Requirements: Plan for your non-fast days! In order not to binge, you'll need to plan ahead, and develop a balanced meal plan to eat moderately and snack on low-carb treats on so-called "feast" days. Despite the name, an element of "feast day" discipline is required, or all is for naught. While you can indulge in a real treat occasionally, temper your cravings in order to see results.

Cooking and shopping: Essentially, you can continue your regular cooking and shopping, as long as you stick to healthy foods that have low or no simple carbohydrates.

Can I use packaged food and meals?: No. Absolutely not, No way, no how. See the Keto section for more information as to why prepared foods are *verboten*.

Are there in-person meetings to attend?: None necessary, although partnering with a friend is highly recommended for mutual support. There are no weigh-ins or rah-rah sessions.

Exercise: How much you exercise is up to you. But obviously, you're not going to have a lot of energy for that on your fasting days. The creators of the Every Other Day diet studied people doing cardiovascular exercise (like biking, walking, running, or dancing) while on the alternate-day fasting plan and found that they were able to maintain muscle mass while fasting.

<u>Does IF follow restrictions/allow for preferences?</u>: Since you are free to choose what food and food quantities you eat, IF can work with any food restrictions -- whether vegan or vegetarian, a meat eater, prefer high- or low-carb foods, want to avoid certain fats, etcetera. But note that you could have side effects like fatigue, feel weak at times, and have headaches, since your caloric intake will ideally be reduced.

Here are some other considerations you should know:

<u>Are there additional costs?</u>: None beyond your regular shopping. Actually, your grocery bills should decrease, because you'll eat much less on those 2 to 4 days per week you'll be fasting. A ketogenic/healthy foods shopping list is at the end of this eBook.

<u>Is there support?</u>: Books and websites exist detailing variations on intermittent fasting, but there's no single website for fasting support, However you'll find Keto diet resources online that are helpful once you've decided which IF fasting plan works best for you.

<u>Final Tips</u>: Most intermittent fasting information recommends cutting back to 500-600 calories on fasting days. Many people may find this both medically safer for people on medications that must be taken with meals. And at least at first, such low-calorie intake will prove easier than not eating at all fast days.

Remember to drink enough clear fluids on fast days to prevent dehydration. And you'll need a healthy eating plan for days that you don't fast.

<u>Does it work?</u>

- Several studies assessing intermittent fasting diets show at least short-term weight loss after following your fast and feast routine for several weeks. Be aware that overeating on non-fast days can be your downfall.

- Will the weight loss will last over a longer time? That's not clear with any diet, or form of calorie restriction, my dear. The duration of the results is up to you,

- Why cut back every day if you can drop pounds by watching what you eat only a couple of days a week? That's the logic behind intermittent fasting, and a reason it is becoming more popular in recent years.

- There are different versions of intermittent fasting; the general idea for each plan is that you eat normally some days of the week and drastically reduce calories on other days.

- Some plans encourage you to skip food entirely for a maximum of 24 or 36 hours at a time. Others, such as the Every-Other-Day plan or the 5:2-Fast=Diet, allow you to have some food but assure that you only get about one fourth of your regular calories.

Are there other effects? In some studies, people who followed this diet did lose weight *and* also had a decrease in some inflammation markers. Fasting puts your cells under mild stress, and scientists think the process of responding to this stress, on your low-calorie or full fast days, strengthens your cells' ability to deal with stress and potentially fight off or control some diseases.

How Long Can / Should a Person Fast?

Most water-only fasts last 24 to 72 hours. You should not follow a water-only fast for longer than this without medical supervision.

Apparently, the world record for fasting is 382 days (although we don't recommend this!), and going 7-14 days may be possible for some people. One danger of fasting longer than 14 days is a perilous mineral/fluid shift called refeeding syndrome that occurs when food is reintroduced after an extremely long fast.

Humans Were Made to Eat Intermittently

Our bodies are made to adjust to periods of feast or famine. Our earliest ancestors were nomadic and opportunistic hunter-gatherers who grew no crops and stored no food but instead feasted on seasonal fruits, nuts and greens, or stuffed themselves after a large kill, in anticipation of being forced to go without when the season, the weather, or changes in climate so dictated. It has been said that the migration of early man was undertaken in pursuit of food sources. As the vegetation disappeared and the animals moved on in search of edible plants and small creatures, humans followed their primary food source.

Voluntarily going without food is not known to have been practiced when food was scarce. Since those with the best chance of long-term survival were those whose bodies were most efficient in storing necessary fat to sustain them though the lean times, people tended to eat to the maximum when seasonal fruits and berries and wild grains were available, drying some naturally, where possible, to eat later. Animal kills were maximized, with all parts of the animal being used – Skins and horns and bones for clothing and implements, and every edible part was eaten.

Feast and famine were the rules of the day, and our eating patterns were far from regular. For hundreds of the seasonality of foods and their limited quantities, plus the great amount of physical labor necessary to complete daily tasks, move about the community and complete daily work ensured that obesity was fairly rare.

Is it any wonder that in this day of abundance and excess, obesity and its corollary illnesses and chronic conditions are becoming a major problem in nations all around the world?

Intermittent fasting

Also known as intermittent energy restriction, intermittent fasting (IF) is an umbrella term for a number of meal timing schedules that alternate between periods of voluntary fasting and non-fasting over a given expanse of time. Non-caloric and sometimes low-caloric drinks (usually referred to as 'clear liquids') can be taken during intermittent fasting, contrary to extremely strict (absolute, or 'dry') fasting in which restrictions even disallow fluid intake, as is often required in religious practices.

A suggestion for anyone interested in adopting a practice of intermittent fasting is to try it for a month to see if an IF schedule works for you. Try a few of the variations to see which one accommodates your normal daily schedule. Before diving in unprepared, start by following a high fat, high protein and low-carbohydrate diet in anticipation of adopting an IF fasting lifestyle. A low-carbohydrate ketogenic (Keto) diet is perfect to use in tandem with intermittent fasting, although other low-carbohydrate diets will also reduce your hunger, retrain your appetite, and so will make intermittent fasting easier. This kind of diet will also prevent you from bingeing on non-fasting days.

Even a low-carb diet may provide a degree of weight loss and type 2 diabetes reversal.

But be aware that if you overeat on your non-fast days, or if you continue eating simple carbohydrates, which readily turn into sugars in your system and provide instant energy, but soon leave you hungry, you may not lose weight with a fasting routine.

Examples of simple carbohydrates include food additives like white and brown sugars, corn syrup, glucose-fructose-sucrose, fruit juice concentrates, and common foods like baked goods, packaged cookies, sugary soda, and most common breakfast cereals.

Complex carbohydrates include fruits, vegetables, whole grains, legumes (beans and peas), oats, potatoes, and so forth. Complex carbohydrates have lots of fiber and are more filling; they take longer to digest and so satisfy hunger longer than simple carbs do.

Intermittent fasting is pattern of eating, and *not* a diet, per se. With IF you are making a conscious decision to intentionally skip meals entirely (or partially) on pre-determined days, or only eat within an 8-hour time frame, and fast the other 16 hours every day. IF does not depend on calorie counting or continuous calorie reduction. Within reason, and by eliminating simple carbohydrates, you can eat pretty much wheat you want. Bacon and eggs? Go for it! Ditch the cereal and choose this breakfast. Want a grilled steak with a side of mushrooms in butter, a baked potato, and creamed spinach? You've got it. Skip the rolls, ditch the desert, and enjoy.

While there are a variety of methods to implement intermittent fasting, the different eating schedules that can be employed on an ongoing basis share a single concept: You eat normally during non-fasting periods but stick to a specific time frame for ingesting food, and fast over identified, planned days, or during certain hours of the day, and overnight.

Some types of intermittent fasting diets are flexible and, rather than totally abstaining from all but water and clear, non-caloric fluids on fast days, suggest that you cut back instead to consuming just 500-600 calories. For diabetics, and people fasting while under a doctor's care, or those who are on medications that must be taken before or after meals, this particular pattern is easier and medically safer than total abstinence. It you have any kind of medical condition, always consult a physician before starting any kind of diet, heavy exercise, or fasting routine.

Intermittent fasting effectively mimics out ancestral eating patterns. They did not have means of preserving foods beyond drying and salting, or keeping foods in cool cellars for as long as possible before decay and rot set in – and, in fact, costly spices from the countries to the east were prized by our European ancestors for their ability to disguise the taste of decomposing meats and rotting vegetables.

Through much of the world's history, people would cycle through often extended periods of famine, punctuated by periods of feasting, when crops were plentiful, and hunts were productive. There were no grocery stores or 24-hour markets, refrigerators or freezers. In fact, even into the early 20th century, refrigerators powered by electricity were rare, and blocks of ice were regularly to delivered to middle-class homes to keep foods cool.

Our bodies are more accustomed to deprivation than plenty, to hard work and walking long distances rather than a sedentary lifestyle and occasional workout at the gym.

Around the world, and especially in the United States, obesity is reaching a crisis, and combined with lack of exercise, is responsible for many of our diseases.

Going without food, or fasting, as it turns out, provides many health benefits. Modern research is providing indisputable evidence that cycling through alternate periods of feasting and fasting actually results in biochemical benefits through the alteration of the way in which our bodies operate.

The early hygienists and naturopathic hllollowers of Natural Cure philosophy of medical practice were wiser than they knew. Today's researchers are providing definitive evidence that the disease process is driven not just by eating too much, but by eating too often.

When your body is constantly in "feast mode" and we are programmed to eat three times a day, whether it is hunger that prompts us to the eat or just habit, the normal physical processes of natural repair and rejuvenation are short-circuited. Our bodies are naturally programmed for periodic repair and maintenance, which it forgoes when energies and organs are focused on the biochemical processes involved with digestion and storage of sugars, fats and nutrients,

Animal studies repeatedly demonstrate that severe caloric restriction does indeed promote weight loss; but it also extends longevity. While "starvation dieting" is not an enticing for people accustomed to eating at will and "pigging out" on holidays, or when depressed and disappointed in ourselves or our lives, the good news is that research also shows you can achieve most (if not all) of those starvation benefits and recreating a "feast or famine" scenario by simply restricting daily calorie intake through intermittent fasting.

WHAT HAPPENS TO YOUR BODY AND BRAIN WHEN YOU FAST?

Many health field professionals and practitioners are actively promoting the amazing health benefits and increased cognitive function that result from fasting as a lifestyle choice. Although fasting is an ancient health tool, successfully practiced for centuries for religious reasons, people still question its legitimacy as a cure for the ills of aging, and for specific diseases that plague modern man such as cancer and diabetes. Some even question whether fasting is a legitimate means to maintaining good health.

Some people equate fasting with self-starvation and question its value. This is readily countered by countless anecdotal evidence to the contrary, which shows that fasting has instead, health benefits that virtually anyone can achieve through routine practice.

Your brain goes into survival mode when you fast, increasing your ability to better focus on tasks at hand. Fasting has also been shown to reduce oxidative stress, and reduce inflammation, insulin resistance and blood sugar levels - all of which are good for the brain health and function. IF also reduces the varied risks of metabolic syndrome, which is not of itself a disease, but is a cluster factors that can raise your risk of heart disease, cardiovascular disease and stroke, as well as type 2 diabetes. The symptoms and risk factors posed by metabolic syndrome include

- High blood pressure

- High blood sugar

- High cholesterol

- Overweight and difficulty in losing weight due to insulin resistance

- Abdominal fat; large waist circumference

It has long been known that dietary changes have an effect on the human brain, and in fact, those who study childhood epilepsy are aware that children who suffer epileptic seizures have fewer of them when placed on a calorie restrictive diet or begin a routine of fasting. It has further been observed by researchers that such children do show improved seizure control when placed on a high fat and low-carbohydrate diet, along the lines of what is known as a ketogenic or Keto diet.

The theory is that fasting aids the brain in taking protective measures to counteract the over-excited signaling the epileptic brain generally exhibits that can trigger seizure activity.

The evolution of the human brain – including the higher cortical functions– has been driven by the need to sustain optimal levels of cognitive performance while in a fasting, or food-deprived state.

The most effective means of shedding unwanted pounds, intermittent fasting is also the most effective way to eliminate sugar cravings. When sugar is no longer your body's primary fuel, you'll not crave it when your stores of sugar run low.

Last, but far from least, intermittent fasting acts as a potent ally to prevent and possibly even treat dementia. Ketones are released as a byproduct of fat burning, and ketones (not glucose) are actually your brain's preferred fuel.

HOW LONG SHOULD I FAST INTERMITTENTLY TO OBTAIN THE BEST EFFECTS?

Intermittent fasting is not a diet – it is a pattern of eating that can be sustained for years. Intermittent fasting is lifestyle that can provide a multitude of health, cognitive and longevity benefits, and is most effective when continued indefinitely.

Considering that your blood and nervous system are essential to virtually every bodily function, and to your very physical existence and good health, can you think of a better reason to incorporate intermittent fasting in your life?

WHAT SHOULD I CONSIDER BEFORE I START A FASTING ROUTINE?

If you fail to take into account your current physical state of health, and do not properly research the matter before starting to fast, or when absolute or 'dry' fasts are undertaken without forethought and are continued to excessive lengths, or when such extended fasts are undertaken repeatedly over many years with little respite.

But intermittent fasting, with good hydration during fasts and the consumption of a nutritious diet on days that you do not fast poses no danger at all, and is extremely beneficial.

Not all fasts are suitable or convenient to your particular situation. Therefore, it is wise to prepare yourself by considering your needs and goals, understanding how many calories you should consume, learning how best to fast, reviewing the different time frames that are commonly used for intermittent fasting, and the results one can expect if done properly.

As with a program of strenuous exercise, you should discuss any concerns before embarking on a major lifestyle change, and discuss any health issues with your doctor. If have been diagnosed with cancer, diabetes, neuromuscular disease, cardiovascular disease, have a prescription for a medication that must be taken with meals, or have any congenital problem that might make fasting a serious decision, you should be fasting under the supervision of a physician. Itis likely that he or she will work with you to find an appropriate method of fasting, and may need to monitor your progress.

To facilitate your undertaking, it is a good idea to begin altering what you normally eat and look into adopting alternative dietary models as Keto, Atkins or other low carbohydrate, high fat diets with no processed food or simple carbohydrates permitted. These made aid in a transition to the discipline and regimes required for successful fasting.

By starting such a diet in preparation for beginning a regimen of intermittent fasting, you will wean yourself off sugars and begin burning fat as a source of energy, which will diminish sugar cravings and leave you feeling fuller after meals, since simple carbs are burned quickly for energy and hunger quickly returns. The diets mentioned feature foods that are high in fiber, which is filling, and protein takes longer to digest than carbohydrates do; plus. Fats are necessary for good neural functioning.

Note that the fasting protocols presented are done by scientists and experts who published thee studies and are well known and respected in their fields. Fasting to achieve these results must be done under the supervision of a knowledgeable physician who is a specialist in the diseases you are interested in ameliorating or reversing, as many of these efforts are still considered experimental, with no promise of success.

Those Who Should Never Fast & Those Who Can, With a Doctor

If you are interested in fasting a few times a week, on alternating days, or simply wish to delay the intake of nourishment for a number of hours to attain the health benefits of a fasting regimen, many physicians aware of the research on fasting would recommend intermittent fasting (IF).

There are, however, a number of people who should absolutely avoid fasting, including:

- Children and individuals under the age of 20

- People living with constant stress (adrenal fatigue)

- Individuals with cortisol dysregulation.

- Women who are pregnant and/or nursing, or who plan to become pregnant in the near future

- Individuals who are underweight for their age, sex and height

- Individuals with eating disorders such as anorexia, bulimia, or other eating disorders, whether they have been medically diagnosed or not

- People with uncontrolled or 'brittle' diabetes

- Individuals with gout or high levels of uric acid

- Those with a serious medical condition such as liver disease, heart disease or kidney disease.

If you're hypoglycemic or a Type 2 diabetic, you should be extra cautious. Those people who use insulin, glipizide, or other diabetes drugs should be supervised by their doctor if they're following IF. Avoiding snacks or skipping breakfast can end badly for diabetics since they need to eat at consistent times to prevent spikes in blood sugar and to increase the effectiveness of the medication they use.

Characterized by abnormally low level of blood sugar, hypoglycemia is associated with diabetes (although you can be hypoglycemic even if not diabetic).

A hypoglycemic crash can include symptoms like headache, weakness, tremors, hunger and irritability. As blood glucose levels continue to plummet, severe symptoms may set in:

- Visual disturbances, such as double vision and blurred vision

- Confusion and/or abnormal behavior

- Seizures

- Loss of consciousness; potential coma

The best way to reduce of eliminate the risk of hypoglycemia is to *eliminate sugars* from your diet, especially fructose and corn syrup, which is often an ingredient in many of the canned goods, prepared foods and baked goods we buy. Eliminating grains, and replacing them with larger portions of quality proteins and healthy fats in a whole foods, low-carbohydrate, high fat diet (like the ketogenic or Keto diet detailed later in this book) will start shifting your body from burning carbohydrates for fuel, which are used up rapidly, leaving you hungry and out of sorts, to burning fat.

Please see your dotor for additional information and answers to questions about utilizing an intermediate fasting program to improve both Type 1 and Type 2 diabetic health. Be sure to start your moderate fasting plan with your doctor's knowledge and permission. Therapeutic diets for improvement of specific diseases or chronic conditions should be conducted under the supervision of your doctor.

Clean your cabinets and fridge: toss or give away processed and canned and baked goods and shop for whole foods. A ketogenic (Keto) list of recommended foods is at the back of the book, along with a number of websites where you can learn more about utilizing a Keto diet and can find recipes and daily menus, plus ideas for snacks.

Coconut oil can help solve some of the issues you may face. It's a rapidly metabolized fat that can be uses as a substitute for sugar, on and in many foods; and since it does not require insulin, it can be used during your fast. Where there is a will, there's a way!

It will take some time for your blood sugar to normalize, whether or not you are diabetic. Sugar cravings - in fact, all carb cravings will gradually lessen and disappear. You'll want to continue paying careful attention to any hypoglycemic signs and symptoms. If you suspect that you might be crashing, be sure to eat something, like a tablespoon of coconut oil. Avoid fasting if you're hypoglycemic, and before starting any fasts, work on improving your overall diet by adopting a whole food LCHF, Keto or Atkins diet (the three are LCHF diets are essentially the same) and normalize your blood sugar levels *first*. Then try out one of the less rigid versions of fasting and the eating and fasting windows that best accommodate your normal schedule.

Individuals on prescribed medications that must be taken with meals should contact their doctors for recommendations as to fasting times. And ask if the medication can be taken with a spoonful of pleasant tasting coconut oil rather than a full meal. And people who take blood pressure medications for heart disease should also check with a doctor when thinking about intermittent fasting.

With proper medical supervision, and determination on your part, you will find there are workarounds for many situations that on the surface, would seem to negate any possibility for you to safely engage in an intermittent fasting routine.

Where there is a will, there's a way!

Start Slowly and Work Up to Changes in Your Dietary Habits

Here are some suggestions on how to start intermittent fasting when you are thinking - possibly – about giving it a try. If your health is compromised in any way, you should consult a physician before starting your first fast. You will want to make sure that fasting won't affect any medications you may be taking or be detrimental otherwise.

If you are younger and have no health concerns, you may prefer to consult a dietician or nutritionist rather than a doctor to help you determine which IF plan would be easiest for you to follow on a regular basis.

When you are ready to start a program in intermittent fasting, you will find that the following advice applies to *anyone* starting a regimen of intermittent fasting, and especially to diabetics. It is advisable for everyone to consult their physician when you have one or more health conditions that could either be worsened or could improve after fasting.

Adopting a Keto or other type of LCHF (low carb high fat) diet will prepare your body to delay food intake without causing a problem with developing hypoglycemia. An LCHF diet will naturally lower your blood sugar, since carbs are immediately processed into glucose by your digestive system and are immediately metabolized into glucose. As your body becomes accustomed to fewer simple carbohydrates (sugars and syrups, processed foods, and baked goods, sweets, popular cereals and so forth), and your meals include more vegetable fiber and protein, vegetable and animal fats, your sugar levels will decrease, affecting insulin needs, if you are a diabetic.

Why is it important to change your diet *before* starting a fasting routine? You want to make the fasting experience and tolerable and easy to comply with as possible. If you have weaned yourself from the simple carbohydrates that comprise a great part of the American diet of today, carbs that are metabolized as quick-burning sugar, not only will weight lost be more achievable, but you will have fewer problems with hunger, and with fluctuations in blood sugar; you will be better able to fight the temptation to cheat, will have a greater ability to consistently stick with it, and follow the eating schedule you have chosen over a long term in order to achieve the full benefits, and will suffer few of the initial side effects that are cause b the physical adjustments to calorie restriction.

Just by following the low-carb, high fat diet of your choice, you will begin seeing and feeling the difference - appreciating the positive changes in what you weigh and how you feel.

Only when your body has accommodated the dietary changes and has made the major adjustment in shifting to burning fat as fuel, will you be ready to add intermittent fasting to the mix, and select the IF fasting program that will best suit your daily schedule.

What Makes Intermittent Fasting the Best Choice? Facts About Intermittent Fasting

- **<u>Simplicity – and a single schedule</u>: You** needn't worry about what or how much you're permitted to eat, count calories, keep track of "points," or weigh in publicly – and pay for the privilege of embarrassing yourself! Instead, you just concentrate on your fasting schedule.

- **<u>Meals will taste better</u>**: When you're not constantly, hunger hormones aren't released as frequently and your body develops better hormonal balance, enabling you to better control your appetite.

- **<u>Cravings for sugary, fatty foods won't torment you</u>**: Your sweet tooth will subside, and you'll find it easier to quit late-night snacking habits because IF forces you to stop eating at a certain time. Beneficially, those who crave foods high in refined carbs and sugar will find they have more control over this behavior, as a keto diet shifts the body's energy fuel from carbs to fats. Desire for chips and high-calorie snacks will decrease and you'll find that you naturally avoiding snack-filled aisles when grocery shopping.

- **<u>You'll renew cells in a whole-body anti-aging process</u>**: Intermediate fasting (IF) kick-starts increased production of human growth hormone (HGH), which research has shown promotes improved cellular repair. Not eating for several consecutive hours creates slight stress on cells' mitochondria, nudging them to "clean house" and eliminate depleted cells, thus revving up your overall cellular functioning.

- **If you're prediabetic, IF can help get sugar under control:** If you've been diagnosed with the symptoms of metabolic syndrome and are developing insulin resistance, and potential Type 2 diabetes, as your doctor if fasting intermittently is worth a try. This type of eating plan and a Keto diet will help your cells become more sensitive to insulin. When you eat, your body releases a hormone, insulin, to move sugar from your bloodstream to your cells for energy. People who are prediabetic have insulin resistance, which means cells in your body have decreased responsiveness to insulin. When they take up glucose, it remains in your blood, and your blood sugar levels stay elevated. Intermittent eating requires your body to pump out insulin less often. IF has been shown to improve insulin sensitivity.

- **IF helps when weight loss efforts have plateaued:** Intermittent fasting may operate to kick-start your metabolism.

- **You will reduce cancer risks:** Research studies have demonstrated that IF can help lower your risk of cancer because fasting leads to apoptosis, or programmed cell death. After a certain number of divisions, our cells are programmed to die. Apoptosis, or programmed cell death, is one of the primary mechanisms utilized in targeted cancer treatment. With apoptosis, your body has more consistent cellular turnover, thus preventing the potential for abnormal cells to develop into cancer.

Methods of Intermittent Fasting (IF): What They are and How They Work

Are you okay with skipping morning breakfast? Do you prefer a.m. work outs, and to forgo dinner? Do you eat out a lot and have an active social life, filled with frequent gatherings that involve eating and drinking with friends? Do you have an Aunt Angelina who is a marvelous cook and often invites you to dinner (or lives with you), constantly urging you to, "Mangia, mangia!" ? ("Eat, eat!")

You'll have to experiment with the eating and fasting intervals that work best for you. And you will need to convince friends and family that your periodic fasts will not cause you to wither away in front of their eyes.

Many problems can be resolved by scheduling such encounters on your "feast" days, and exercising moderation at table. Or starting your daily 'eating window' late in the day. so that dinnertime is accommodated.

Referring your family to websites that explain intermittent fasting in lay terms may quiet their concerns. But, as many reformed alcoholics can attest, there is tremendous social pressure from others to "Just have one drink," and who hasn't been encouraged to "Try just a little piece of the cake." When this happens, you can claim no appetite, or use the old "I just ate" excuse. But there will inevitably be occasions that will become problematic when one fasts. Intermittent fasting is still poorly understood by many.

And, as with virtually all restrictive diets, there are drawbacks. For some people who are sensitive to caffeine, drinking caffeinated drinks while fasting can disrupt their circadian rhythm, and thereby, their metabolism. Challenges do exist.

Thankfully, IF is an umbrella term which encompasses a wide variety of fasting schedules. Essentially, IF is an eating pattern that cuts calorie consumption – entirely or in part – by refraining from eating and from drinking caloric beverages for a certain number of hours within each day, or on specified days.

There are at least six schedules for intermittent fasting that have become popular, and while they may popularly go by different names, with mild variations, the essential timetables are :

- **<u>The 5:2 Plan:</u>** Fast 2 days a week, with daily caloric intake of 500 (women) and 600 calories (men). Since the calorie limit is separated by a 10 to 12-hour fast, half the calories are consumed in the morning and the other half in the evening. OR you can undertake a 24-hour fast twice a week (or just once weekly), a plan that is popularly dubbed, 'Eat-Stop-Eat.'

- **<u>Alternate-Day Fasting</u>:** Fast every other day, using the same calorie limits as the 5:2 Plan, but do this every other day of the week rather than just two days weekly. Including time asleep, each fast can last 32-36 hours. The drawback? You go to sleep on an empty stomach every other night. An important "however" is that this fasting schedule boasts a higher compliance rate than many of the other IF schedules, and is much easier to maintain over the long run.

- **<u>The Warrior Diet</u>**: Under eat for 20 hours during night and day, then eat a single huge meal in the evening. Boiled eggs, legumes, yogurt, raw fruit/veggies and legumes can be eaten on rising and at midday, as well as small amounts of dairy. Drinking plenty of non-caloric, clear beverages and water is recommended. The Warrior Diet is the brain-child of Ori Hofmeckler, a soldier in the Israeli Special Forces and is intended to emulate the diet of ancient warriors, who were on the move or fighting during the day', and only had the time and a situation suitable to preparing and eating a major meal when they encamped at night.

- **<u>Longer Fasts: 24-hour/One-Meal-a-Day and the 36-hour Water Fast</u>:** Some people find that fasts permitting small meals totaling only 500-600 calories, with the suggestion to apportion the calorie total into two small meals simply does not work for them, since the small meals prompt hunger sensations that encourage them to forage in the fridge for more to eat.

Water fasts encourage you to fill up with water when you feel you must eat. It is interesting that when you take on absolute fasts with water, tea or black coffee being the only permitted beverages, your body becomes adjusted to the total absence of food for a number of hours at a time, and you do not feel hungry. Furthermore, hunger pangs tend to come in waves, so when your stomach begins rumbling, reach for your glass or bottle of water. Fill up on water and it will pass.

Fasters often prefer longer fasts for that reason. A 24-hour or 36-hour fast can generally be undertaken once, twice, or three times a week.

A 24- or 36-hour fast is not as grueling as it sounds, when you recognize that sleep will take up many of those hours. A 24-hour fast takes you from breakfast, lunch or dinner on one day to that same time the next, with eight hours for sleep. Note that in a 24-hour fast, even if it is a water fast, you will still consume one meal each of the two days covered by the fast. This is actually identical to the **One-Meal-a-Day** schedule.

Your 36-hour fast will be slightly different: You will fast one entire day, plus six hours or less on the first and the third days. Here is how that works: You eat your dinner on Day 1 at 7:00 p.m. for example, skip *all* meals on Day 2, and then eat again when you have a normal breakfast at 7 a.m. on day 3. So that is a total of 36 hours of fasting. With 16 hours of sleep on the two night of the fast, that will equate to a waking fast of around 20 hours over the three days.

- easier to maintain with Keto.

Fats, as opposed to carbohydrates, are a slow-burning fuel to create energy you need for your body to function properly. Because it burns so slowly, you can keep going on less food for a longer period of time without the dramatic and disconcerting sugar fluctuations and energy crashes carbs evoke in most individuals, as with the "donut highs" and energy wipe-outs that result from an overload of carbohydrates. And once your body adjusts to change, you'll be amazed at how your cravings disappear and how you can go for many more hours without even thinking of food. Your insulin and leptin resistance improve, along with your weight and cholesterol levels, blood pressure and sugar control. You will find late-night snacking urges have vanished and that you will tend not to eat anything for up to four hours before bedtime, which is beneficial for those with hiatal hernias or acid reflux, and results in better sleep. You'll be surprised how you will be satisfied with far less food and still feel sated,

During periods of fasting, be certain that you are drinking enough fluids, sticking with water, unsweetened tea and black coffee. Drinking lots of water will not only help you stay hydrated, but it will help you eliminate waste products in your system, reduce hunger, still cravings and avoid muscle cramping and headaches that can be caused by dehydration. It is also crucial to eat high-quality, high-nutrition foods when you do eat.

How Should I Decide on the Best IF Fasting Method for Me?

Ultimately, the best fasting schedule is one you'll be able to comply with, week after week. If you find yourself repeatedly cheating, skipping days, shortening fast windows or actually forgetting your fasting schedule, intermittent fasting won't work.

You may need to experiment with different IF schedules to find one that works for you. The key is to find an approach that you are confident you can sustain over the long run.

The Side Effects of Intermittent Fasting

Like most diets, intermittent fasting has side effects. They can be unpleasant, but most are temporary, as your system adjusts. Aside from **headaches** (mitigate by taking salt), **constipation** (use a common laxative if uncomfortable), **muscle cramps** (drink more water), **heart burn** (use an antacid) and **hunger** (this will pass), you may be:

Feeling fatigued or tired, and irritated

When you skip meals, your blood sugar naturally drops, and that may affect your mood and your energy levels. Glucose is the primary energy source for brain function, and when not consuming the number of calories to which your body is accustomed, your disposition may sour. Headaches are common and feelings of irritation can make you less pleasant to be around, and that can also keep you from wanting to be social or exercise and work out.

You may feel fatigued or lacking in energy, even when you are not tired.

One thing you can do to prevent severe drops in energy levels is to pay attention to your diet on non-fast days and times, eating more fiber- and protein-rich meals with healthy fats. Load up on lean protein like grilled chicken or salmon, grass-fed beef, and use eggs in a variety of dishes. Plant-based options include edamame, chickpeas, and quinoa, they'll fill both protein and fiber needs. Add healthy fats like avocado and nuts to help you feel more satiated.

Plan your "feast day" meals and use a list to shop from until you know the foods you need and want. After a time on a ketogenic diet, you will find yourself avoiding the central aisles at the grocery store that hold simple carbohydrate snacks, canned goods, sugared cereals, processed foods, desert mixes and the like. Pack your own lunch to take to work or on field trips, or when you travel.

Adequate hydration is crucial, and you will need more fluids when you fast, as well as before and after, since a good deal of our daily fluid requirements are met by the foods that we eat. We often confuse thirst with hunger, eating when we should be hydrating.

Feeling dizzy or lightheaded

Going long hours without food, can cause dizziness, and feelings of being lightheaded. Lightheadedness might a symptom of hypoglycemia, a condition signifying very low blood sugar. Other common symptoms of hypoglycemia include shakiness, sweating, fatigue, and irregular heartbeat. Should you be you're prone to hypoglycemia and follow an intermittent fating schedule. Carefully monitor your symptoms, and fast under the supervision registered dietitian, or a doctor or to avoid big dips in your blood sugar

What You Can Eat on 'Keto'...

A ketogenic diet is recommended,

- High in healthy fats. Many will benefit from 50-85 percent of their daily calories in the form of healthy fat from avocadoes, organic grass-fed butter, pastured egg yolks, coconut oil, and raw nuts such as macadamia, pecans, and pine nuts

- Moderate amounts of high-quality protein from organically raised, grass-fed or pastured animals. Most will likely not need more than 40 to 70 grams of protein per day

- Unrestricted amounts of fresh vegetables, ideally organic.

During fasting periods, drink copious amounts of water, unsweetened tea with no milk or cream, black coffee, and you can even indulge in an *occasional* diet soda, although unsweetened, effervescent soda water is preferable.

On days when you don't fast, you can eat pretty much whatever you want. But to shed pounds and get the nutrients you'll require, you should stick to healthy whole foods.

On fasting days, you'll eat very little food or nothing at all.

And What You Can't...

You should absolutely avoid processed and canned foods with hidden sugars and salt, most packaged foods – especially baked goods and other foods filled with simple carbohydrates like sweeteners such as sugars, corn syrup, molasses, honey and syrup, most candies, cookies, sweet treats and desserts, breads, pastas, beer and prepared foods with unlabeled ingredients, as well as potatoes, corn, rice most peanut butters, fruits and concentrated fruit juices.

WHAT IS A KETOGENIC (KETO) DIET, AND WHAT ARE THE BENEFITS?

You have to understand that our bodies have two complementary systems for fueling our bodies and providing the energy necessary for its function. The easiest accessible fuel is glycogen – a fast-burning fuel with limited storage. When the body fuels itself with glycogen, the fuel is quickly used up, causing hunger and continuous eating once the fuel is depleted. The other system is a kind of 'deep storage' with almost unlimited storage space: our body fat. It is difficult for the body to access, unless there are no carbohydrates in the system to burn. Then, perforce, fat is burned as an energy source.

Either way, the energy produced is accessed by your cells through the production of insulin, which ensures your cells are fed.

A 'Keto' or ketogenic diet is a low-carb, high-fat diet that when consumed consistently, will shift your metabolism from burning carbohydrates to burning fat to meet energy needs, and accomplish this in a relatively short period of time, if followed faithfully. And Keto is easy to follow, because as your body adjusts to the change, your cravings will vanish, your appetite will stabilize, and you will feel sated after meals and snacks. Hunger will only return when your body needs more fuel.

Paired with intermittent fasting, eating a Keto diet during your "feast" portion of the 'feast or famine cycle' our bodies were built for, provides a great many benefits,

Keto can have multiple benefits, including rapid weight loss, and improved health and system performance. In addition, Keto is a whole-foods diet that comes highly recommended by a large number of doctors. It is particularly effective for losing body fat while satisfying hunger, and it will also lower blood sugar in everyone who follows it - including Type 2 diabetes. In a Keto diet, you will eat a higher proportion of foods with fat, moderate amounts of protein, and lots of fibrous vegetables.

When combined with an intermittent diet plan that is followed conscientiously under medical supervision, a ketogenic diet has actually been documented to actually reverse Type 2 diabetes in a number of patients.

The Different Types of Keto Diets:

The ketogenic diet has become quite popular under the shortened title, 'Keto.' But it is not a new concept – or a new diet. There have been, of course, very slight but minimal variations in how the various ketogenic diets are employed, and the names of the diets are, of course, different but the diets are essentially the same. But these three (and others

The Keto diet was once known as **'The Air Force Diet'** and was developed by the United States Air Force to keep pilots slim and mentally sharp. It evolved into **'The Atkins Diet'** when its effectiveness was discovered by a cardiologist name Robert Coleman Atkins, and heavily promoted in his book, and its following promotion informed many Americans of the cardiac benefits of a low carb-high fat diet. Then the **'Paleo'** diet came along, followed by **'Keto'** - which is actually named for the process that makes this kind of diet so effective, popular, and relatively easy to follow.

Furthermore, there are several types beyond the popularized diets mentioned above, and these are:

- **The Standard Ketogenic Diet (SKD):** A highly low-carbohydrate, moderate protein and high fat diet that is typically comprised of 75% fat, 20% protein and just 5% complex carbohydrates (vegetables)

- **The Cyclical Ketogenic Diet (CKD)**: This particular ketogenic diet involves specific periods f high carbohydrate 'refeeds' and consists of five (5) ketogenic days followed with two (2) days that are high in carbohydrates

- The Targeted Ketogenic Diet (TKD): Specifically for those who work out regularly and strenuously, larger amounts of carbohydrates are added around workout times.

- The High Protein Ketogenic Diet (HPKD): Similar to the normal ketogenic diet, or 'Keto,' this diet includes a larger amount of protein, with ratios of 60% fat, 35% protein, and only 5% carbs

Benefits Unrelated to the Different Types of Keto Diets:

As mentioned, any kind of ketogenic diet will serve to provide certain benefits, regardless of which specific type of ketogenic diet you choose to follow:

- Healthier food choices

- Weight loss

- Lower blood sugar

- Improved ability to think clearly

- Increased energy and physical endurance after adjusting to the regimen

Benefits Unrelated to Health Issues:

- Improved cognitive function, mental clarity and concentration

- More time on fast days, when meal preparation is nil

- More time on "feast" days, when less food is required, reducing preparation time

- Better physical appearance for both women and men

- Aids bodybuilders to build lean muscle without relying on complicated eating rules or the need to constantly eat small portions of food through the day

- Appetite Control

What truly makes these diets different is the extent and manner in which these diets have been researched, and the number of studies undertaken that have resulted in extensive information related to the astounding medical benefits of a ketogenic diet, particularly when undertaken in tandem with one of the many scheduled eating plans known as 'intermittent fasting.' Only the Keto diet has been directly studied extensively when combined with a program of intermittent fasting.

WHAT ARE POSSIBLE HEALTH BENEFITS WHEN ADOPTING A KETOGENIC 'KETO' DIET, APART FROM A FASTING ROUTINE?

Results of studies on ketogenic diets that don't incorporate fasting tell us...

- **How Keto Affects Symptoms of Metabolic Syndrome:** A number of studies demonstrate that low-carb ketogenic diets like Keto significantly reduce several risk factors for developing heart disease by improving your cholesterol profile, raising high density lipoprotein (HDL) and modestly lowering your low-density lipoprotein (LDL) or 'bad' cholesterol and your total cholesterol levels. It reduces blood sugar levels, improves insulin sensitivity, and reduces blood pressure – all the symptoms of metabolic syndrome and insulin resistance. Reversing the symptoms of metabolic syndrome greatly reduces your likelihood of developing cardiovascular and heart disease.

- **How Keto Affects Diabetes:** A ketogenic diet, even undertaken without fasting, reduces and stabilizes blood sugar levels, increases insulin sensitivity, and can potentially reduce or eliminate dependence on Type 2 diabetes medications, and slightly reduce required dosages of injected insulin for Type1 diabetics. The metabolized, simple carbs found in breads, cakes and desserts, sweets and sweeteners, starchy foods and candies are sugar machines, overproducing fuel faster than it can be expended, thus raising blood sugar levels. Low-carb diets that include only complex carbs found in vegetables and other healthy foods solve that problem, leading to significant weight loss, which is related to reversing Type 2 diabetes. And one study found the Keto diet increased insulin sensitivity by an amazing 75%!

- **How Keto Affects Cancer:** In cancers, too, abnormal cells feed on sugars. By reducing blood sugar levels considerably, a ketogenic diet will help to starve cancer cells of needed sugars to fuel abnormal cellular growth. The Keto diet is being currently employed to slow tumor growth and treat several types of cancer, and in particular, breast cancer.

- **How Keto Affects Epilepsy:** The ketogenic diet is a proven and often effective medical therapy for epilepsy that has been in use since the 1920s. It was primarily used to treat the condition and massively reduce epileptic seizures in children. More recently, it has been found that epileptic adults have shown benefits from a Keto diet, as well. When on a Keto diet, some individuals have been able to reduce their use of anti-seizure medications and still remain free of seizures. This can reduce the severe side effects of seizure medication, when taken for long periods of time, and in quantities sufficient to control seizures. The studies also show increased mental performance when on a Keto diet, due to better seizure control, since every seizure inflicts a degree of damage to the brain.

- **How Keto Affects Alzheimer Disease:** The high fat content of a Keto diet is truly brain food, and fat is necessary for your synapses to properly transmit messages to nerves and muscles, to regulate the motor functions of your limbs and to support your cognitive abilities whenever you think. learn and speak. Studies indicate that, once again, the high fat content of a ketogenic (Keto) diet improves brain function, and suggest that a Keto diet may actually reduce symptoms of Alzheimer's disease, slowing its progression.

- **How Keto Affects Autism:** For whatever reasons, the incidence of children who show symptoms in varying degrees that place them on the autism spectrum has increased dramatically in recent years. Research is showing that these children can benefit greatly from the high fat content of a Keto diet, improving cognitive function, concentration, verbal abilities, learning abilities, and significantly helping with behavioral issues that can characterized the affliction.

9 HEALTH IMPACTS ON CHRONIC CONDITIONS MERITING FURTHER RESEARCH

1. **Parkinson's disease:** One study found the Keto diet helped improve symptoms of Parkinson's disease.

2. **Polycystic ovary syndrome:** A ketogenic (Keto) diet can help reduce insulin levels, which possibly play a key role in polycystic ovary syndrome

3. **Severe Acne:** Lowering insulin levels plus eating less sugar, simple carbs and processed foods may contribute to improving acne, lessening unwanted outbreaks.

4. **Traumatic Brain Injuries:** One promising animal study found that the Keto diet can reduce concussions, aiding recovery after brain injury, but only if the ketogenic diet is initiated immediately after the injury.

5. **Glycogen Storage Disease:** Typically, diagnosed in childhood, people with glycogen storage disease (GSD) lack one of several enzymes that help store glucose (blood sugar) as glycogen, or break glycogen down into glucose. Symptoms can

include poor growth, low blood sugar, muscle cramps, fatigue, and an enlarged liver. Early research suggests a ketogenic diet may benefit some forms of GSD.

6. **Nonalcoholic Fatty Liver Disease (NAFLD):** The most common liver disease in the Western world is nonalcoholic fatty liver disease (NAFLD). It is strongly associated with Type 2 diabetes, obesity, and metabolic syndrome. It is strongly linked to type 2 diabetes, metabolic syndrome and obesity, and there's evidence this condition improves with adherence to a very low-carbohydrate ketogenic (Keto) diet.

7. **Migraine Headaches:** Typically, migraine headaches involve severe pain, nausea and sensitivity to light. Studies suggest migraine symptoms often improve in those who adopt Keto diets, with reduction in frequency and medication needed for relief.

8. **Multiple Sclerosis (MS):** MS damages the myelin sheath, the protective envelope surrounding nerve fibers. That leads to a host of communication problems between brain and body. MS is a degenerative disease with symptoms including numbness and problems with balance, movement, vision and memory, with gradual loss of all function. MS appears to involve a reduction in the cells' ability to use sugar as a fuel, like most nerve diseases, and studies have pointed to the potential of a strict Keto diet to suppress inflammation, assist with cell repair and energy production, reduce other disease markers, and improve quality of life for MS patients.

9. **GLUT1 Deficiency Syndrome:** Glucose transporter 1 (GLUT1) deficiency syndrome is a rare genetic disorder. Symptoms begin following a child's birth and can include developmental delays, seizures, and movement difficulties. A Keto diet may help because – unlike glucose – ketones do not require this particular protein to cross the blood/brain barrier. A ketogenic diet can provide an alternative course to fuel the brains of these children.

A Shopping List for Beginners - Foods for a Keto diet

Cheeses:

American Bleu Cheese Cheddar Cottage Cheese

Cream Cheese Feta Gouda Mozzarella

Parmesan Provolone Ricotta Cheese Swiss Cheese

Dressings:

Red Wine Vinegar/Olive Oil Bleu Cheese Creamy Caesar Ranch

Fats & Oils:

Almond Butter Avocado Oil Butter Cocoa Butter Coconut Oil

Flax Seed Oil Grape Seed Oil Fish Oil Hemp Seed Oil MCT Oil

Macadamia Oil Full Fat Mayonnaise Olive Oil Walnut Oil

Seeds:

Chia Flax Hemp Pumpkin Safflower Sesame Sunflower

Nuts & Legumes:

Almonds Brazil Nuts Coconut Hazelnut Macadamias Pistachios

Pecans Walnuts

Seafood:

Anchovies Bass Carp Flounder Haddock Halibut Mackerel Sole

Sardines Tilapia Trout Tuna Clams Crab Lobster Mussels

Oysters Shrimp Squid

Flours, Meals & Powders:

Acorn Flour Almond Flour Almond Meal Cocoa Powder Coconut
Flour

Flax Seed Meal Protein Powder Psyllium Husk Sesame   Seed
Flour Splenda

Eggs, Poultry & Fowl:

Eggs Chicken Duck Goose Quail Turkey

Fruits & Berries:

Avocado Blackberry Blueberry Cranberry Lemon Lime

Green Olive Raspberry Strawberry Rhubarb Tomato

Dairy & Dairy Substitutes:

Almond Milk (Unsweetened) Coconut Cream Coconut Milk
(Unsweetened) Greek

Yogurt Heavy Cream Sour Cream (Full Fat) Soy Milk
(Unsweetened)

Whipped Cream Grass Fed Butter

Meat:

Beef Tongue Beef Ribs Beef Roast Pastrami Beef Sausage Corned Beef

Ground Beef (70%-90% Lean) Beef Tenderloin Beef Hot Dogs/Frankfurters Steak

Bologna Lamb Pepperoni Pork Bacon Pork Chops Ham Liverwurst

Braunschweiger Pork Loin Pork Roast Pork Tenderloin Veal Venison

Vegetables:

Arugula Asparagus Bok Choy Broccoli Broccoli Rabe Cabbage Cauliflower

Celery Chard Chicory Greens Cucumber Eggplant Endive Fennel Green Beans

Jalapeño Lettuce Parsley Radishes Spinach Soy Beans Zucchini

HOW WILL MY BODY REACT TO KETO DIETARY CHANGES + FASTING?

It's true that a fat-burning ketogenic (Keto) diet will be beneficial to your weight loss efforts, and general health, as will be adopting a new eating pattern of intermittent fasting.

However, know that any major dietary change will initiate several strange and unexpected effects on your body, until your system adjusts to the new regimen. Be forewarned.

Bad breath, increased urination, and what is affectionately called the 'keto flu' are keto are Keto setbacks to look out for, along with feeling faint and weak, dizziness, headaches, muscle cramping and general fatigue prompted by fasting – as was addressed in the earlier chapters on intermittent fasting.

These physical reactions occur during the adjustment period of both dietary modification, which are departures from your normal eating habits, That is why this book recommends preparing for intermittent fasting by first changing your diet to a low-carb, high fat mode of eating, and allowing your system to adjust to a Keto diet before taking a second leap into a full-blown intermittent fasting regimen.

A staged preparation will make the effects far milder than attempting both changes in unison. You will not be so uncomfortable, disoriented and physically overwhelmed that you simply figure you cannot handle it any longer, and quit your attempt at self-improvement.

The fact that you are reading this book is a wise decision – one that will help you prepare for these major lifestyle changes ahead.

Since people handle change much better when they know what to anticipate, and when they understand that discomforts will pass as your body acclimates to the new routines, you will do much better than many others.

It is important to be mindful of unpleasant complications and know what to expect before you embark on this journey of rebuilding both your physique, and your health. Knowledge will make you strong.

Strong enough to keep pushing through until you get comfortable with these dietary changes - and not quit as you might, if you are taken by surprise.

1. **Your breath will probably smell:** When your body moves into the fat-burning stage of ketosis, ketones released during this process will likely affect the smell of your breath, and cause a weird or almost sweet taste in your mouth. Sugarless breath mints, or chewing anise seed will help.

2. **It is likely you will urinate more:** You will be hydrating more often, and on top of that, a ketogenic diet reduces inflammation in your body, reducing the water that binds with inflammation in your tissues, and the glycogen (sugar) carbs stored in your liver also lead to water retention in your liver, and your muscles. When you urinate mor and more frequently, you are flushing out your system.

3. **The infamous 'Keto Flu" is part of the adjustment process:** Transitioning into a ketosis state as you remain on the Keto diet leaves you feeling as though you've been walloped by a case of the flu. The symptoms are virtually the same. Fortunately, this is a temporary state, and will pass quickly, lasting only two to four days at maximum. Some lucky souls may not experience it at all.

4. **Digestive changes will occur:** Prepare for temporary rumblings, bloating, gas, and potentially explosive change in bowel movements. You will survive.

5. **You may experience cramps:** As you lose the water stored in your organs and tissues, electrolytes may fall out of balance. This ultimately causes cramping. For relief, drink lots of water and take sea salt or drink mineral water to stop the rumbling. And rest. Munch some high mineral nuts or seeds. That will help.

6. **Keto adjustment may mess with your ZZZs:** You may temporarily experience sleep difficulties and your schedule may be disrupted.. Again, mineral-packed foods and lots of water will go to work to set you right.

7. **Once you've hit ketosis, you'll feel MAH-VE-LOUS!:** You'll find yourself filled with energy, your libido will awaken, and all the restorative and antioxidant effects will kick in, leaving you wondering why you waited so long to try this!

8. **Your thyroid function may improve:** As your body begins to work more efficiently its ma become more efficient, metabolically speaking. If you are taking medications, you may want to visit your physician to see if dosages should be recalibrated.

9. **Your bones may need more minerals:** In initial ketosis, your body will be producing more acid, and that should be neutralized by taking a one-a-day mineral supplement.

CONCLUSION

Congratulations!

You've reached the end of this eBook introduction to intermittent fasting (IF) and ketogenic (Keto) dieting, and now you are prepared to change your life for the better.

Keep this as a guidebook to your journey, and check out the online sources mentioned. Click the links included in the online version to learn still more; to access more of the scientific information; and watch several of the informative videos to meet the leading doctors in the field and hear them speak.

Don't forget to wander through the internet for resources from which to choose recipes, meal plans, and Keto snacks you might enjoy. They will surely help you make your diet simply delish!!!

Plan your first grocery shopping trip, and don't forget to photocopy and take the Keto shopping list with you!

Remember that you will have help in your dietary travels through the forests of information and over tossing seas of doubt and possible discomfort. You will be introduced to sweeping new ideas, share information with others about their own Keto and IF experiences, and encounter medical jargon about dry studies and startling research results that you may find confusing, wondering which and how these growing numbers of findings might apply to you.

If information becomes overwhelming, remember that you have many guides who are just a mouse click away.

Bon voyage!!

www.ingramcontent.com/pod-product-compliance
Lightning Source LLC
Chambersburg PA
CBHW050659250726

48662CB00002B/759